Contents

- Introduction 2
- Scene Survey 2
- Casualty Assessment 3
- Basic Life Support 7
- Shock 16
- Fainting 18
- Bleeding and Wounds 19
- Head Injuries 26
- Eye Injuries 28
- Nosebleeds 31
- Dental Injuries 31
- Chest Injuries 33
- Abdominal Injuries 34
- Blisters 35
- Swallowed Poison 36
- Insect Stings 37
- Tick Removal 39
- Thermal Burns 42
- Chemical Burns 44
- Electrical Injuries 45
- Frostbite 47
- Hypothermia 48
- Heat-related Emergencies 48
- Fractures 50
- Spinal Injuries 53
- Muscle Injuries 54
- Heart Attack 55
- Stroke 57
- Diabetic Emergencies 58
- Convulsion 59
- Emergency Delivery of a Baby 61

Introduction

First aid is the immediate care given to an injured or suddenly ill person. First aid does not take the place of proper medical treatment. It consists only of furnishing temporary assistance until competent medical care, *if needed,* is obtained, or until the chance for recovery without medical care is assured. *Most injuries and illnesses require only first aid care.*

Scene Survey

The first step in any emergency situation is to do a scene survey. The following guidelines apply in most cases:
1. Take charge of the situation.
2. Shout for help to attract bystanders.
3. Scan for hazards. If the scene is unsafe, make it safe. If you are unable to make the scene safe, do not enter.
4. Determine the number of casualties.
5. Determine the likely cause of the injury or nature of the illness for each casualty.
6. Identify yourself as a first aider. Offer to help and obtain consent.

Casualty Assessment

After sizing up an emergency situation initially and deciding if it is safe to provide first aid for the casualty there, the first aider can then find out what is wrong and how serious it is by following a systematic approach known as *casualty assessment*.

Casualty assessment of an injured or an ill person consists of:
- Initial check
- Physical examination and SAMPLE history

Initial Check

The initial check covers these areas in this order:
  Airway open?
  Breathing normal?
  Severe bleeding?

The initial check finds and corrects life-threatening conditions.

Airway. Ask yourself: does the casualty have an open airway?

If the casualty can talk or is responsive, the airway is open. Refer to page 8 for the correct and detailed procedures for opening the airway of an unresponsive casualty. Take proper precautions if a spine injury is suspected. Refer to page 53 for spine injury care.

Breathing. Ask yourself: is the casualty breathing? Responsive casualties are breathing, but look for any breathing difficulties or unusual breathing sounds. For an unresponsive casualty, keep the airway open and *look* for the chest to rise and fall, *listen* for breathing, and *feel* for air coming out of the casualty's nose and mouth. See pages 8–9 for the correct and detailed procedures for providing CPR.

Severe Bleeding. Ask yourself: is the casualty bleeding heavily? Check for severe bleeding by looking over the casualty's entire body for blood-soaked clothing.

Physical Examination and SAMPLE History

Having completed the initial check and attended to any life-threatening problems, take a closer look at the casualty to discover problems that do *not* immediately threaten life but may do so if they remain uncorrected.

Physical Examination

Check the casualty from head to toe.

Head and Neck. Check the scalp for bleeding or deformity ("egg" or depression). Do *not* move the head during this procedure. Check the ears and nose for a clear fluid or bloody discharge. Look in the mouth for blood or foreign materials.

Eyes. Notice whether pupils are constricted or dilated. Cover the eyes then uncover to see if the pupils react. Look for unequal pupils, since a difference in their size almost always means a medical emergency (Figure 1).

Chest. Check the chest for cuts, bruises, penetrations, and embedded objects.

CASUALTY ASSESSMENT

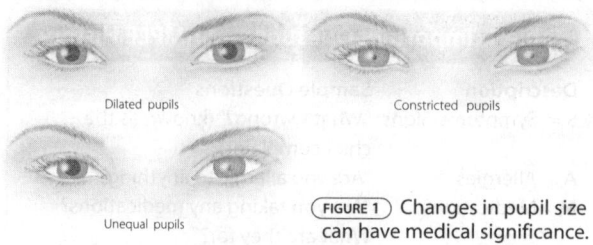

FIGURE 1 Changes in pupil size can have medical significance.

Abdomen. Check for penetrating objects and protruding organs. Ask the casualty to point to where it hurts.

Extremity Assessment. Check the arms and legs by feeling and looking for injury, deformity, and tenderness. Compare one side of the body with the other.

Back. In casualties with possible spinal injury as well as those with suspected stroke, check sensation and strength in all extremities by having them press a foot against your hand and having them squeeze your hand with theirs.

SAMPLE History

Important information about the casualty's condition can be collected from the casualty, and possibly family members, by following a simple questioning technique known as the SAMPLE history (Table 1). Also look for a medical alert tag, worn as a necklace or bracelet, that may identify a casualty's problem.

Chain of Survival

Away from the hospital environment, survival from cardiac arrest depends on four key links, referred to as the

Table 1 Important Questions—SAMPLE History

Description	Sample Questions
S = Symptoms/Signs	"What's wrong?" (known as the chief complaint)
A = Allergies	"Are you allergic to anything?"
M = Medications	"Are you taking any medications? What are they for?"
P = Past medical history	"Have you had this problem before? Do you have other medical problems?"
L = Last oral intake	"When did you last eat or drink anything? What was it?"
E = Event leading up to the illness or injury	Injury: "How did you get hurt?" Illness: "What led to this problem?"

chain of survival (Figure 2). A delay in any of the four links occurring will reduce the effectiveness of any resuscitation attempt and the subsequent chance of the casualty surviving. The four links are:
1. Early access: recognising cardiac arrest and calling 999 (summoning the ambulance service), which are the first and most important steps.
2. Early CPR: good quality CPR supplies a minimal amount of oxygenated blood to the heart and brain; it buys time until a defibrillator is available.

BASIC LIFE SUPPORT 7

3. Early defibrillation: as soon as an AED is attached it will analyse the problem and administer a shock to help restore a normal heart rhythm in some casualties.
4. Early advanced care: trained ambulance service clinicians will be able to continue from the platform set above and administer drugs, further shocks, and more definitive airway procedures.

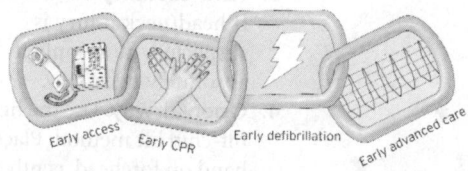

FIGURE 2 Chain of survival.

Basic Life Support

Basic Life Support (BLS) is the second link in the chain of survival. Performed correctly, it sustains a non-breathing casualty or a cardiac arrest casualty with cardiopulmonary resuscitation (CPR). *Cardio* refers to the heart and *pulmonary* to the lungs. Cardiac arrest casualties have a better chance of surviving if CPR is started within 4 minutes of the cardiac arrest, and advanced cardiac life support is received within 8 minutes of the heart stopping.

Adult CPR

If you see a collapsed person ...

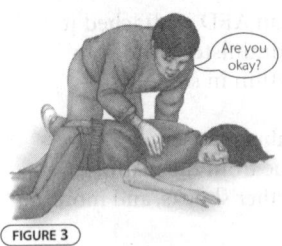

FIGURE 3

1. **Check responsiveness** by gently shaking the casualty and asking loudly, "Are you okay?" (Figure 3)
2. **Shout for help** if no response.
3. **Turn casualty onto back.** If head/neck injury is suspected, move only if absolutely necessary.
4. **Open airway.** Use the head tilt-chin lift method. Place one hand on forehead, gently tilting head back whilst lifting the chin with fingers of the other hand.
5. **Check for breathing.** Put your ear to casualty's mouth/nose, and feel for air movement on your cheek, look for chest movement, and listen for breath sounds. Check for no more than 10 seconds (Figure 4).

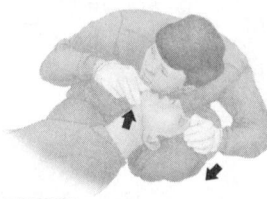

FIGURE 4

Initial steps of cardiopulmonary resuscitation.
FIGURE 3 Determining unresponsiveness.
FIGURE 4 Open airway and check for breathing.

6. If casualty is not breathing send for or **go for help**. On returning, **start chest compressions**. Place the heel of one hand in the centre of the casualty's chest; and place the heel of the other hand on top of the first. Using both hands, give 30 compressions pushing the sternum straight down to 4 to 5 cm. Release pressure on the chest after each compression. The rate of speed must be equivalent to 100 per minute (Figure 5).

BASIC LIFE SUPPORT 9

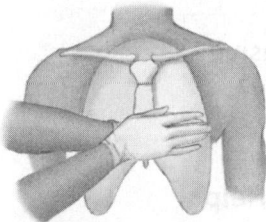

FIGURE 5 Proper hand placement for chest compressions.

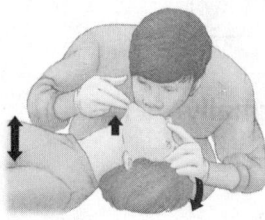

FIGURE 6 Give 2 normal breaths.

7. **Give rescue breaths and chest compressions.** After every 30 compressions, open the airway and give 2 rescue breaths, enough to make the chest rise (Figure 6). If the chest does not rise, re-tilt the head and try another breath. If still unsuccessful, suspect choking and use appropriate procedures found later in this guide.

8. **Do not interrupt resuscitation**, unless the casualty starts to breathe, qualified help arrives, or you become exhausted.

Choking in Adults and Children Over 1 Year Old

Choking occurs when the upper airway becomes blocked and the casualty cannot breathe.

How to recognise choking:
It is important to ask the conscious casualty, "Are you choking?"

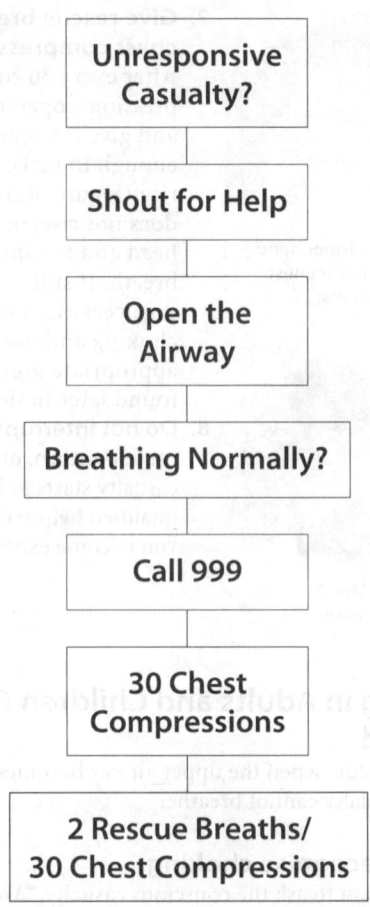

Adult CPR

BASIC LIFE SUPPORT 11

Mild airway obstruction:
- Good—response to question, yes, indicated by coughing forcefully by responsive casualty.
- Poor—response to question, either unable to speak or nods, indicated by weak, ineffective cough; high-pitched noise; blue, grey, or ashen skin, lips, and under fingernails.

Severe airway obstruction:
- Unable to speak, breathe, or cough
- Clutches neck with one or both hands (known as the "universal distress signal for choking")
- Unresponsiveness

First Aid for Responsive Choking Adult:
If casualty is responsive and cannot speak, breathe, or cough . . .

Give up to 5 back slaps, stand to the side and slightly behind the casualty while supporting them to lean forward, and give up to 5 sharp blows between the shoulder blades with the heel of one hand. Check after each blow for success. If the obstruction remains . . .

Give up to 5 abdominal thrusts, stand behind casualty and wrap your arms around casualty's waist. Make fist with one hand and place it just above casualty's navel and well below the tip of the breastbone with the knuckles up. Grasp fist with your other hand. Press fist into casualty's abdomen with sharp, upward thrusts. Each thrust should be a separate and distinct effort to dislodge object. If the obstruction remains . . .

Continue alternating 5 back slaps with 5 abdominal thrusts until the obstruction is coughed out, the casualty starts to breathe or cough, other trained help arrives, or the casualty becomes unconscious.

First Aid for Unresponsive Choking Adult:
If the casualty becomes unconscious, support them carefully to the ground. Immediately call for an ambulance.

Begin CPR. Each time you open the airway to give rescue breaths, look for any objects in the throat. If possible, remove them.

Child Basic Life Support
Basic Life Support for a child between 1 and puberty is similar to that for an adult, with these exceptions:

- In an unwitnessed arrest, summon the ambulance service after 1 minute of resuscitation (for witnessed arrests or adults, summon immediately).

- If the child is not breathing, give 5 rescue breaths, each about 1 to 1.5 seconds long, and watch for chest rise and fall. Reposition child's head to ensure good air entry.

- Look for signs of circulation, such as movement, coughing, etc.

- If there are no signs of circulation, commence chest compressions.

- Compress the lower third of the sternum, one finger's breadth up from the point where the ribs meet.

BASIC LIFE SUPPORT 13

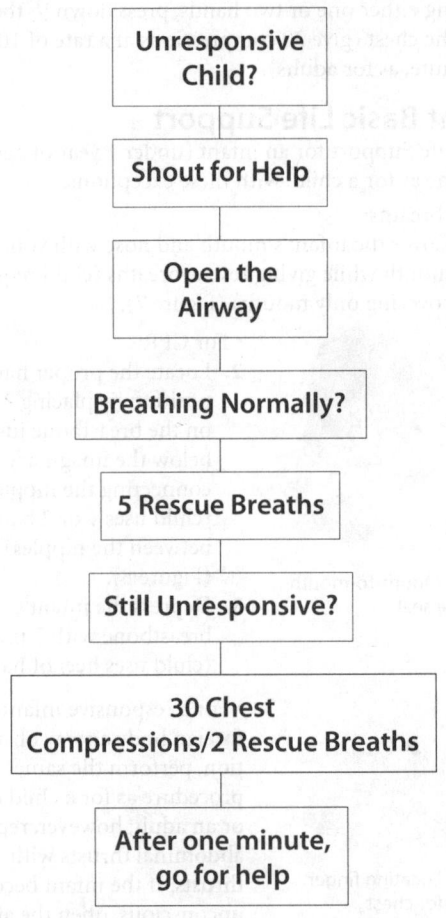

Child CPR

- Using either one or two hands, press down ⅓ the depth of the chest (give 30 compressions at a rate of 100 per minute, as for adults).

Infant Basic Life Support

Basic Life Support for an infant (under 1 year of age) is the same as for a child, with these exceptions:

- For breaths:
  1. Cover the infant's mouth and nose with your mouth while giving rescue breaths (child requires covering only mouth) (Figure 7).

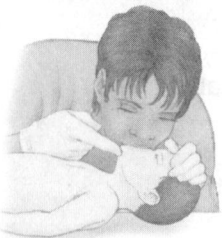

FIGURE 7 Mouth-to-mouth-and-nose seal.

- For CPR:
  2. Locate the proper hand position by placing 2 fingers on the breastbone just below the imaginary line connecting the nipples (child uses 1 or 2 hands between the nipples) (Figure 8).
  3. Depress the infant's breastbone with 2 fingers (child uses heel of hand).

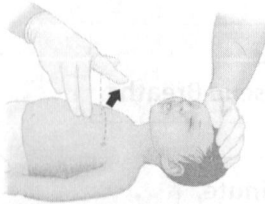

FIGURE 8 Locating finger position for chest compressions in infant.

- For a responsive infant with a foreign body airway obstruction, perform the same procedure as for a child over 1 or an adult; however, replace 5 abdominal thrusts with 5 chest thrusts. If the infant becomes unconscious, open the airway, attempt 5 breaths, and commence CPR.

AED

Once you have determined the need for an AED (casualty not breathing and unresponsive), the basic operation of all AED models for anyone over 1 year of age follows this sequence:

1. Perform CPR whilst someone goes for the AED and calls 999. If you are alone, you will have to do this yourself.
2. Once the AED is available, turn the equipment on.
3. Apply the electrode pads to the casualty's bare chest and the cable to the AED. Use child pads for a child, if available.
4. Stand clear and analyse the heart rhythm.
5. Deliver a shock if indicated.
6. Immediately resume CPR at 30:2 (2 minutes).
7. Check the casualty and repeat the analysis, shock, and CPR steps as needed.

Recovery Position

If an unconscious patient is breathing and has not suffered trauma, the best way to keep the airway open is to place the patient in the recovery position (Figure 9). The recovery position helps to keep the patient's airway open by allowing secretions to drain out of the mouth, instead of back into their throat. It also uses gravity to help keep the patient's tongue and lower jaw from blocking the airway.

To place a patient in the recovery position, carefully roll the patient onto one side as a unit without twisting the body. You will achieve greatest leverage by flexing the patient's leg that is furthest away and pulling it towards yourself. You can use the patient's hand to help hold their head in the proper position. Place the patient's face on its

POLICE FIRST AID POCKET GUIDE

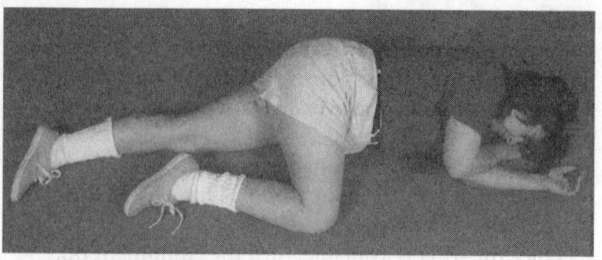

FIGURE 9 Recovery position.

side so any secretions drain out of the mouth. The head should be in a position similar to the tilted back position of the head tilt-chin lift technique.

Recovery Position for Suspected Spinal Injuries

If a spinal injury is suspected and the casualty remains unconscious, the above technique should be modified, using two people to turn the casualty. The first person should hold and steady the head whilst another rolls the casualty. The casualty's back should be maintained in-line as much as possible; using another one or two people will help control the roll.

Shock

Treat all injured casualties for shock.
- Care for life-threatening injuries and other severe injuries.

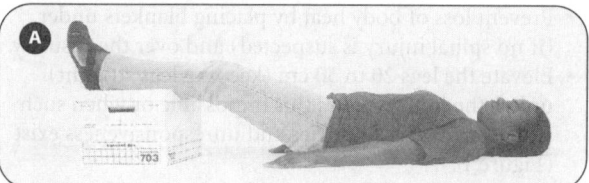
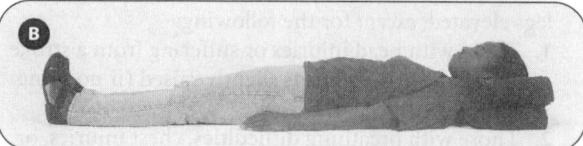
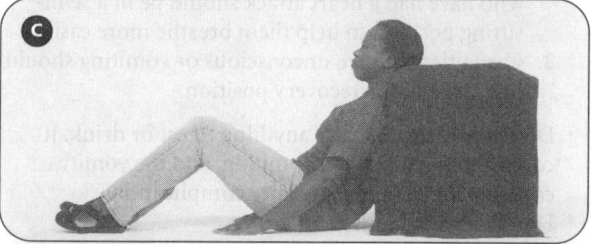
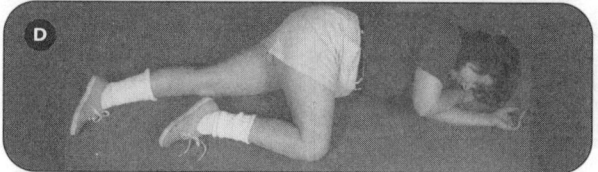

FIGURE 10 A–D) Positions for shock. **A.** Elevate the feet and legs 20 to 30 cm for most situations. **B.** Casualties with head injuries should have their heads slightly raised (if no spine injury is suspected). **C.** If the casualty is having breathing difficulties, chest injuries, or a heart attack, then they should be in a semi-sitting position. **D.** If the casualty is unresponsive but breathing, place the casualty on their side.

- Prevent loss of body heat by placing blankets under (if no spinal injury is suspected) and over the casualty.
- Elevate the legs 20 to 30 cm (keeping legs straight) unless the injury makes this impossible or when such situations as chest injuries and unresponsiveness exist (Figure 10).
- Casualties should be kept on their backs with only the legs elevated, *except* for the following:
  1. Those with head injuries or suffering from a stroke should have their heads slightly raised (if no spine injury is suspected).
  2. Those with breathing difficulties, chest injuries, or who have had a heart attack should be in a semi-sitting position to help them breathe more easily.
  3. Casualties who are unconscious or vomiting should be placed in the recovery position.
- Do *not* give the casualty anything to eat or drink. It could cause nausea and vomiting, and the vomitus could be inhaled, causing later complications.
- Handle the casualty very gently.

Fainting

- Lay the casualty down and elevate the legs 20 to 30 cm.
- If vomiting begins, turn the casualty on their side to keep the airway open and clear.
- Loosen tight clothing.
- If the casualty has fallen, look for injuries.
- Wet a cloth with cool water and wipe the casualty's face.

- Do *not* splash or pour water on the casualty's face.
- Do *not* use smelling salts or ammonia inhalants.
- Do *not* slap the casualty's face as an attempt to revive him or her.
- Do *not* give the casualty anything to drink until he or she has fully recovered.

Most fainting cases are not serious, and the casualty usually regains consciousness quickly. Seek medical care if the casualty does not regain consciousness within 2 minutes, or remains drowsy for more than 5 minutes.

Bleeding and Wounds

Blood coming from a wound usually stops after 5 to 10 minutes with proper first aid.

- Remove any clothing covering the wound.
- Protect against infection by wearing medical examination gloves or using other methods of protection (eg, extra layers of dressings, plastic material).
- Control bleeding by using the following methods *in order*, until bleeding stops:
  1. *Direct pressure.* Most external bleeding can be controlled by direct pressure over the wound. Steps in applying direct pressure:
     - Place a sterile gauze dressing or any available clean cloth directly over the wound and press against it.
     - Apply a pressure bandage over the gauze dressing to free yourself to attend to other

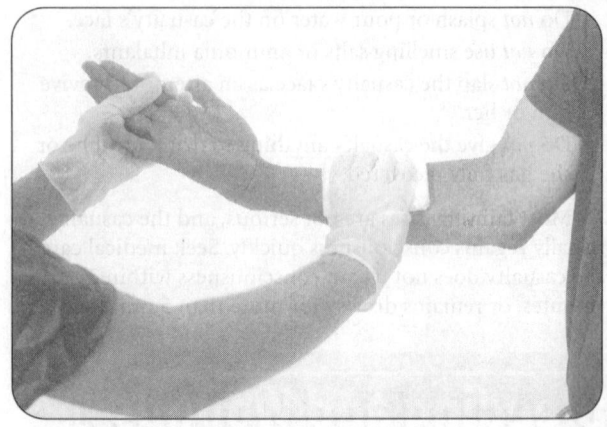

FIGURE 11 Applying direct pressure to a wound.

injuries. The dressing is best held in place with a roller bandage wrapped tightly over the dressing and above and below the wound site.
- Do *not* remove a dressing after placement because bleeding may start again. If a dressing becomes blood-soaked, apply another dressing on top of it and hold them both in place.
- If bleeding does not stop, apply more pressure.
- After bleeding has stopped, maintain pressure with a bandage (Figure 11).

2. *Elevation*. If bleeding persists, continue applying direct pressure and elevate the extremity above the heart level. Elevation alone will not stop bleeding.
3. *Pressure points*. If bleeding continues, apply pressure at a pressure point whilst applying direct pressure

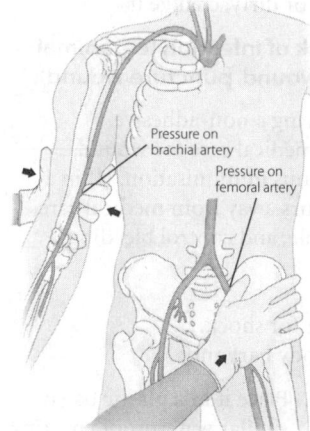

FIGURE 12 Proper hand positions for applying pressure on the femoral and brachial pressure points.

on the wound. A wound may be supplied by more than one major bleeding vessel, so using the pressure point alone will rarely control severe bleeding. Use the brachial point in the arm and the femoral point in the groin. Using pressure points requires a skillful, knowledgeable first aider. Unless you know the exact location of the pulse point, the pressure point technique is useless (Figure 12).

- Do *not* remove a penetrating object.
- Save amputated part(s) by using the procedures shown on page 22.

For shallow wounds (not usually seen by a health care professional):

- Wash the wound with soap and water.
- Cover the wound with a sterile gauze dressing and bandage.

- If a dressing becomes wet or dirty, change it.

For wounds with a high risk of infection (eg, animal bite, very dirty or ragged wound, puncture wound):

- Prevent infection by applying a non-adhesive, absorbent dressing. Seek medical care for wound cleaning and possible tetanus immunisation. (If in a remote location many hours away from medical care, clean the wound, if possible, and control bleeding.)

Amputations

- Control bleeding and care for shock.
- Recover the amputated body part and:

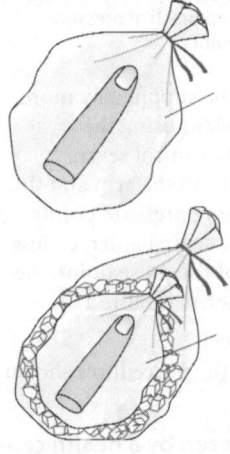

FIGURE 13 Care of an amputated part.

1. Place it in a plastic bag or similar waterproof covering (medical glove, cling film, etc.).
2. Gently wrap the bagged part in gauze or light cloth. This is intended to keep the part away from immediate contact with ice.
3. Keep the bagged, wrapped part dry and cold. Placing the package in a container of ice is okay, but do not let the part become frozen (Figure 13).

- If the injured part is still partially attached by a

Adult CPR

If you see a collapsed person ...

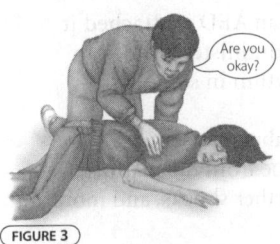

FIGURE 3

1. **Check responsiveness** by gently shaking the casualty and asking loudly, "Are you okay?" (Figure 3)
2. **Shout for help** if no response.
3. **Turn casualty onto back.** If head/neck injury is suspected, move only if absolutely necessary.
4. **Open airway.** Use the head tilt-chin lift method. Place one hand on forehead, gently tilting head back whilst lifting the chin with fingers of the other hand.

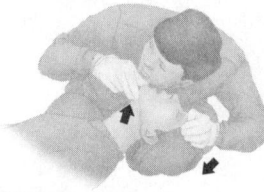

FIGURE 4

Initial steps of cardiopulmonary resuscitation.
FIGURE 3 Determining unresponsiveness.
FIGURE 4 Open airway and check for breathing.

5. **Check for breathing.** Put your ear to casualty's mouth/nose, and feel for air movement on your cheek, look for chest movement, and listen for breath sounds. Check for no more than 10 seconds (Figure 4).
6. If casualty is not breathing send for or **go for help**. On returning, **start chest compressions**. Place the heel of one hand in the centre of the casualty's chest; and place the heel of the other hand on top of the first. Using both hands, give 30 compressions pushing the sternum straight down to 4 to 5 cm. Release pressure on the chest after each compression. The rate of speed must be equivalent to 100 per minute (Figure 5).

BASIC LIFE SUPPORT

3. **Early defibrillation:** as soon as an AED is attached it will analyse the problem and administer a shock to help restore a normal heart rhythm in some casualties.
4. **Early advanced care:** trained ambulance service clinicians will be able to continue from the platform set above and administer drugs, further shocks, and more definitive airway procedures.

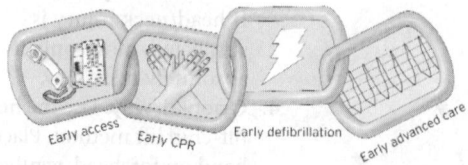

FIGURE 2 Chain of survival.

Basic Life Support

Basic Life Support (BLS) is the second link in the chain of survival. Performed correctly, it sustains a non-breathing casualty or a cardiac arrest casualty with cardiopulmonary resuscitation (CPR). *Cardio* refers to the heart and *pulmonary* to the lungs. Cardiac arrest casualties have a better chance of surviving if CPR is started within 4 minutes of the cardiac arrest, and advanced cardiac life support is received within 8 minutes of the heart stopping.

Table 1 Important Questions—SAMPLE History

Description	Sample Questions
S = Symptoms/Signs	"What's wrong?" (known as the chief complaint)
A = Allergies	"Are you allergic to anything?"
M = Medications	"Are you taking any medications? What are they for?"
P = Past medical history	"Have you had this problem before? Do you have other medical problems?"
L = Last oral intake	"When did you last eat or drink anything? What was it?"
E = Event leading up to the illness or injury	Injury: "How did you get hurt?" Illness: "What led to this problem?"

chain of survival (Figure 2). A delay in any of the four links occurring will reduce the effectiveness of any resuscitation attempt and the subsequent chance of the casualty surviving. The four links are:

1. Early access: recognising cardiac arrest and calling 999 (summoning the ambulance service), which are the first and most important steps.
2. Early CPR: good quality CPR supplies a minimal amount of oxygenated blood to the heart and brain; it buys time until a defibrillator is available.

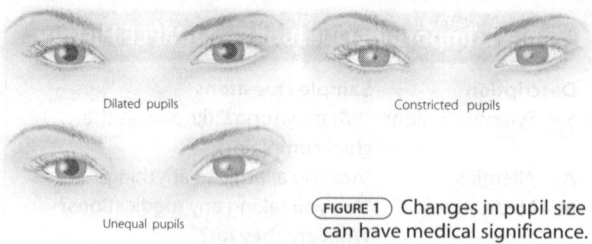

Dilated pupils

Constricted pupils

Unequal pupils

FIGURE 1 Changes in pupil size can have medical significance.

Abdomen. Check for penetrating objects and protruding organs. Ask the casualty to point to where it hurts.

Extremity Assessment. Check the arms and legs by feeling and looking for injury, deformity, and tenderness. Compare one side of the body with the other.

Back. In casualties with possible spinal injury as well as those with suspected stroke, check sensation and strength in all extremities by having them press a foot against your hand and having them squeeze your hand with theirs.

SAMPLE History

Important information about the casualty's condition can be collected from the casualty, and possibly family members, by following a simple questioning technique known as the SAMPLE history (Table 1). Also look for a medical alert tag, worn as a necklace or bracelet, that may identify a casualty's problem.

Chain of Survival

Away from the hospital environment, survival from cardiac arrest depends on four key links, referred to as the

Breathing. Ask yourself: is the casualty breathing? Responsive casualties are breathing, but look for any breathing difficulties or unusual breathing sounds. For an unresponsive casualty, keep the airway open and *look* for the chest to rise and fall, *listen* for breathing, and *feel* for air coming out of the casualty's nose and mouth. See pages 8–9 for the correct and detailed procedures for providing CPR.

Severe Bleeding. Ask yourself: is the casualty bleeding heavily? Check for severe bleeding by looking over the casualty's entire body for blood-soaked clothing.

Physical Examination and SAMPLE History

Having completed the initial check and attended to any life-threatening problems, take a closer look at the casualty to discover problems that do *not* immediately threaten life but may do so if they remain uncorrected.

Physical Examination

Check the casualty from head to toe.

Head and Neck. Check the scalp for bleeding or deformity ("egg" or depression). Do *not* move the head during this procedure. Check the ears and nose for a clear fluid or bloody discharge. Look in the mouth for blood or foreign materials.

Eyes. Notice whether pupils are constricted or dilated. Cover the eyes then uncover to see if the pupils react. Look for unequal pupils, since a difference in their size almost always means a medical emergency (Figure 1).

Chest. Check the chest for cuts, bruises, penetrations, and embedded objects.

CASUALTY ASSESSMENT   3

Casualty Assessment

After sizing up an emergency situation initially and deciding if it is safe to provide first aid for the casualty there, the first aider can then find out what is wrong and how serious it is by following a systematic approach known as *casualty assessment*.

Casualty assessment of an injured or an ill person consists of:
- Initial check
- Physical examination and SAMPLE history

Initial Check

The initial check covers these areas in this order:

Airway open?
Breathing normal?
Severe bleeding?

The initial check finds and corrects life-threatening conditions.

Airway. Ask yourself: does the casualty have an open airway?

If the casualty can talk or is responsive, the airway is open. Refer to page 8 for the correct and detailed procedures for opening the airway of an unresponsive casualty. Take proper precautions if a spine injury is suspected. Refer to page 53 for spine injury care.

POLICE FIRST AID POCKET GUIDE

Introduction

First aid is the immediate care given to an injured or suddenly ill person. First aid does not take the place of proper medical treatment. It consists only of furnishing temporary assistance until competent medical care, *if needed,* is obtained, or until the chance for recovery without medical care is assured. *Most injuries and illnesses require only first aid care.*

Scene Survey

The first step in any emergency situation is to do a scene survey. The following guidelines apply in most cases:

1. Take charge of the situation.
2. Shout for help to attract bystanders.
3. Scan for hazards. If the scene is unsafe, make it safe. If you are unable to make the scene safe, do not enter.
4. Determine the number of casualties.
5. Determine the likely cause of the injury or nature of the illness for each casualty.
6. Identify yourself as a first aider. Offer to help and obtain consent.

Contents

Introduction 2
Scene Survey 2
Casualty Assessment 3
Basic Life Support 7
Shock 16
Fainting 18
Bleeding and Wounds 19
Head Injuries 26
Eye Injuries 28
Nosebleeds 31
Dental Injuries 31
Chest Injuries 33
Abdominal Injuries 34
Blisters 35
Swallowed Poison 36
Insect Stings 37
Tick Removal 39

Thermal Burns 42
Chemical Burns 44
Electrical Injuries 45
Frostbite 47
Hypothermia 48
Heat-related Emergencies 48
Fractures 50
Spinal Injuries 53
Muscle Injuries 54
Heart Attack 55
Stroke 57
Diabetic Emergencies 58
Convulsion 59
Emergency Delivery of a Baby 61

Nosebleeds

Most nosebleeds can be stopped by these simple procedures:
- Keep the casualty in a sitting position to reduce blood pressure.
- Keep the casualty's head tilted slightly forward so that the blood can run out the front of the nose, not down the back of the throat, which causes either choking or nausea and vomiting. The vomitus could be inhaled into the lungs.
- Pinch both nostrils together for 5 to 10 minutes. Remind the casualty to breathe through his or her mouth and to spit out any accumulated blood.
- Seek medical care if bleeding does not stop.

Dental Injuries

Objects Wedged between Teeth
- Attempt to remove the object with dental floss. Guide the floss in carefully so the gum tissue is not injured.
- Do *not* use a sharp or pointed tool to remove the object. If unsuccessful, advise the person to go to their dentist or call the out-of-hours helpline.

Bitten Lip or Tongue
- Apply direct pressure to the bleeding area with a sterile gauze or clean cloth.
- For a swollen lip, apply a cold pack.
- Seek medical care if the bleeding persists or if the bite is severe.

Knocked-out Tooth
More than 90% of knocked-out teeth can be saved with the proper treatment.
- For a completely knocked-out tooth, take it, along with the casualty, to a dentist immediately. With proper first aid procedures, the tooth may be successfully re-implanted in the socket.
- Do *not* put the tooth in water, mouthwash, or alcohol, or scrub it with abrasives or chemicals. And do *not* touch the root of the tooth.
- Place the tooth in saliva or cool milk.
- A partially extracted tooth can be pushed back into place without rinsing the tooth. Then seek a dentist so the loose tooth can be stabilised.
- If you are in a remote area with no dentist nearby, replant a knocked-out tooth by first rinsing it with saliva or milk to clean away debris (do *not* scrub the tooth), and then gently repositioning it in the socket, using adjacent teeth as a guide. Push the tooth so the top is even with the adjacent teeth. Successful replanting usually occurs within 30 minutes of the accident. See a dentist as soon as possible.

Broken Tooth
- Clean any dirt, blood, and debris from the injured area with a sterile gauze or clean cloth and warm water.
- Apply a cold compress on the face, next to the injured tooth, to minimise swelling.
- For a suspected jaw fracture, give the casualty some soft padding and advise them to support the area of concern. If they tolerate it, allow them to place a cold pack against the area to help with pain relief.
- Keep the casualty still and ensure that ambulance service clinicians have been called.

Chest Injuries

Rib Fracture
The casualty can point out the injury's exact location. Deep breathing, coughing, or movement may be quite painful. There may be a rib deformity, bruise, laceration, shortness of breath, severe coughing, or coughing up of blood.

Have the casualty hold a pillow or similar soft object against the injured area.

Sucking Chest Wound
Close off this wound quickly with anything available to stop air from entering the chest cavity. The best way is with a piece of plastic taped in place, leaving one side untaped. This creates a flutter valve that prevents air from being trapped in the chest cavity. Do *not* remove an embedded object. This is a life-threatening injury and

requires immediate ambulance service attendance. Make sure an ambulance is en route.

Abdominal Injuries

Severe Blow

A severe blow to the abdomen can cause internal organ bruising and bleeding. Place the casualty on one side in a comfortable position, and prepare for vomiting.

Penetrating Injuries

If there is a penetrating object, leave it in and bandage around it to control external bleeding and to stabilise the object. Do *not* remove the object.

Protruding Organs

If any of the abdominal organs lie outside the abdominal cavity, do *not* try to re-insert them inside the abdomen. Keep any extruding organs moist, warm, and clean with a moist, sterile dressing. Do *not* cover them tightly or with any material that clings or disintegrates when wet (Figure 17).

Seek medical care for all casualties with abdominal injuries.

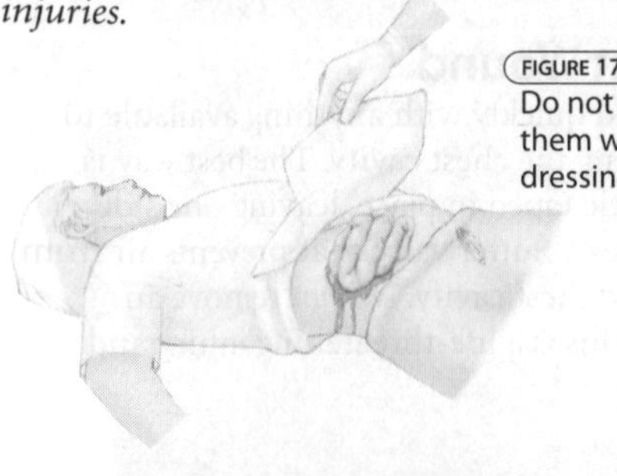

FIGURE 17 Protruding organs. Do not re-insert them. Cover them with a moist, sterile dressing.

Blisters

(This information does *not* apply to blisters from burns, frostbite, or poisonous plants.) To treat a small blister formed by friction, cover it with an adhesive bandage. This will protect the blister from further injury and relieve pain.

A large blister should be covered with a gauze dressing, which allows the area to "breathe," or a stack of gauze pads cut in a doughnut shape to dissipate pressure from the blister. Whenever possible, do *not* break a blister (Figures 18A and B). However, if the pain is unbearable, the blister can be broken and drained.

When a blister must be broken because of pain:

- Wash the area with warm, soapy water and dry thoroughly.
- Make several small holes at the base of the blister with a sterilised needle (Figure 18C).
- Drain the fluid by applying gentle pressure to the blister's top, which should not be removed. In some cases, the blister may have to be drained several times in the first 24 hours. Apply several layers of moleskin or mole foam cut in a doughnut shape on top of each other.
- If a blister is open, wash the area with soap and water to prevent infection. A protective bandage or other cover should be used for 10 to 14 days.
- Check each day for signs of infection (redness or pus). Seek medical care if the blister becomes infected.

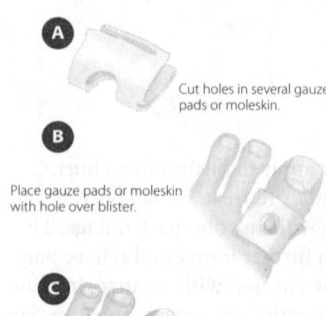

FIGURE 18 A–C Blister care.
A. Unbroken blister. Cut holes in several gauze pads. **B.** Stack the pads on the skin with the holes over the blister. Loosely tape an uncut gauze pad over the top. **C.** If blister is painful or likely to break, use a sterilised needle to puncture the blister's edge.

Cut holes in several gauze pads or moleskin.

Place gauze pads or moleskin with hole over blister.

Do not remove blister's top.

Painful blister can be drained by making small hole with sterilised needle.

Swallowed Poison

Determine the following critical information:
1. *Who? Age and size of the casualty.*
2. *What? Type of poison swallowed.*
3. *How much? How many?*
4. *Why? Accidental or intentional?*
5. *When? How long ago?*
6. *What else? Was anything else taken (alcohol, etc.)?*

- For conscious casualties attempt to find out as many answers to the above questions as you can. Call 999 and ensure qualified help is on the way. Be wary, as some poisons do not produce side effects until hours later, whilst some cause immediate damage.

- Unless advised by ambulance control or another qualified source, do not automatically give water or milk to dilute except when the casualty has swallowed caustic or corrosive substances (eg, acids and alkalis).
- Do not induce vomiting or neutralise unless advised to do so.
- Retain all poison containers, plants, and vomitus to help medical staff identify the poison and prescribe appropriate treatment.
- For an unconscious casualty, whilst ensuring you do not become contaminated, open their airway and check for breathing. Place the casualty in the recovery position on their left side, as this delays stomach emptying into the small intestine. Initiate CPR where appropriate. Call 999 as soon as possible.

Insect Stings

A person who is severely allergic to insect stings can be killed by a single sting within minutes.

Those who have had a reaction to an insect sting should consult with their GP about obtaining a self-administered adrenaline or EpiPen kit and instruction on how to treat themselves so they can protect themselves from severe reactions. They should also be advised to purchase a medical alert bracelet or necklace identifying them as insect-allergic.

- Examine the sting site for a stinger embedded in the skin. If it is still embedded, scrape the sac away cleanly with a hard object such as a driver's license or credit card.
- Wash the sting site thoroughly.

- Apply an ice pack over the sting site to slow absorption of the venom and relieve pain.
- Observe casualties for at least 30 minutes for signs of an allergic reaction (anaphylactic shock). For the highly allergic, a dose of adrenaline is the only effective life-saving treatment. A GP can prescribe an emergency kit that includes a pre-filled syringe of adrenaline or a spring-loaded device that automatically triggers the injection of adrenaline by a quick thrust into the thigh or a large muscle. The spring-loaded device is useful for those reluctant to use a syringe with a visible needle. The allergic person should take the kit whenever going places where stinging insects are found.

Since adrenaline is short-acting, the casualty must be watched carefully for signs of returning anaphylaxis. It is safer to err on the side of caution and call 999 for anyone who has demonstrated anaphylactic symptoms.

Adrenaline should only be given to casualties who are compromised by a severe reaction. It should not be given in anticipation of a reaction following a sting.

Injuries from Exotic Animals

Whilst bites and stings from animals such as spiders, snakes, and scorpions are not commonplace in the UK, these animals will often be kept as pets and exposure to injuries from them may occur.

It may be possible to get advice from the pet owner on how best to treat a bite or sting; however, when unsure of what to do or what type of animal has inflicted the injury, do the following:

- Get the casualty away from the animal, ensuring your own safety at all times.
- Keep the casualty calm. This will help keep their heart rate down and decrease the dispersal rate of any toxin in the bloodstream.
- Immobilise the limb or area that has been bitten.
- Do not apply a tourniquet.
- Do not attempt to suck any poison out.
- Call 999 immediately. If in a remote area, make an attempt to get nearer to help.

Tick Removal

Use the following methods to remove an embedded tick:
1. Use tweezers and grasp the tick as close to the skin surface as possible and gently lift the tick to "tent" the skin. Hold until the tick lets go. Do not twist or jerk the tick, since this may result in incomplete removal.
2. Wash the bite site with soap and water. Apply an ice pack to reduce pain. Keep the area clean.

   Watch for signs of infection or unexplained symptoms (eg, severe headaches, fever, or rash), which may develop up to a month later. If these symptoms appear, seek medical care immediately.

Carbon Monoxide

Carbon monoxide is an invisible, tasteless, odourless, and non-irritating gas.

A complaint of "having the flu" may actually be a sign of carbon monoxide poisoning. Other signs include the following:

- Headache
- Angina (chest pain)
- Nausea and vomiting
- Dizziness and visual changes (blurred or double vision)
- Breathing and cardiac arrest
- Ringing in the ears (tinnitus)
- Muscle weakness
- Unresponsive

For Carbon Monoxide Casualties:

- Immediately remove the casualty from the toxic environment and into fresh air. Give him or her 100% oxygen either in an ambulance or at an A&E department. This improves oxygenation and it also breaks the linkage between the carbon monoxide and the blood.
- For a responsive casualty, seek medical care involving a blood test to determine the level of carbon monoxide.
- For an unresponsive, breathing casualty, place him or her on one side with the head resting on an arm. Loosen tight clothing and maintain temperature.
- Call 999 immediately.

- Check breathing.
- Give CPR if needed.
- Even when only mild symptoms (eg, headache, nausea) appear, seek medical care if carbon monoxide poisoning is suspected.

Incapacitant Spray Exposure

CS incapacitant, pepper, or PAVA spray can all be used as a temporary incapacitant to subdue violent, aggressive, and uncooperative individuals.

Recognition of Exposure:

The chemical reacts with moisture on the skin and mucous membranes of the eyes and respiratory tract, causing a burning sensation and an involuntary shutting of the eyelids.

Other effects can include:
- Continuous tears and secretions from the nose.
- Burning to the inside of the throat and nose.
- Disorientation and dizziness.
- The individual becomes "incapacitated" temporarily.
- In highly concentrated doses, it may induce breathing problems, coughing, sneezing, nausea, and vomiting.

Care for a casualty affected by incapacitant spray:
- Remove casualty from contaminated area–preferably upwind.
- The best treatment is fresh air, particularly with a small breeze–and also time.

- Tell the casualty
  - the effects are temporary
  - the effects will wear off quicker if they follow your instructions
  - to not rub their eyes or skin as this will prolong and enhance effects
  - the effects should wear off within 15 minutes.
- Occasionally irrigation with fresh water helps; however, this should only be undertaken following medical advice and with cold water. Warm/hot water will cause pores to open and allow the chemical to enter the skin.

Thermal Burns

- Stop the burning process. Immediately extinguish clothing fires by having the casualty "drop and roll," by wrapping him or her in a blanket, or by immersing the area in cool water. The choice of procedure may depend on the burning agent.
- Remove smoldering clothing or soak it in cold water. Do not try to remove clothing stuck to the skin; cut around the clothing and do *not* pull on it since further skin damage will result.
- Other types of injury take priority over a burn (except chemical burns). If the casualty's burns are non-chemical, examine him or her for other injuries first, as though the burn did not exist, so as not to miss other life-threatening injuries.
- Burns of the eyes require special care and protection. Rinse them very gently, but with copious amounts of cool, clean water. Pat dry and

cover with a clean, dry dressing. Immediately call 999 or take to medical care.
- Do *not* put any type of ointment, grease, lotion, butter, antiseptic, or home remedies on burned skin. These dressings are unsterile and may lead to infection. They can also seal in heat, resulting in further damage. However, dressings *specifically formulated to reduce the effects of burns* may be used.

Superficial Burns

Signs and symptoms include redness, mild swelling, tenderness, and pain. Hold the affected area under a cold, running tap for 10 minutes or pour cold water from a jug. This will help reduce the pain. Do not allow the casualty to become cold; cool the burn, not the casualty.

Most superficial burns will not need a dressing; however, it is okay to place a non-adhesive, absorbent dressing over the area and hold it in place with a soft, loose-fitting bandage.

Partial-thickness Burns (small area)

Blisters, swelling, weeping of fluids, and pain identify these burns.
- Apply cold as you would for a superficial burn.
- Do not break any blisters.
- After cooling, dress all partial-thickness burns with a non-adhesive, absorbent dressing held in place with a bandage. Check periodically that the bandage is secure but does not become too tight.

- The casualty should be advised to go to hospital if the burn is large or causes them concern.

Full-thickness and Large Partial-thickness Burns

The skin may look leathery, waxy, or pearly grey. It is sometimes charred.

- Ensure the airway is open and check breathing. Initiate CPR if necessary.
- Treat for shock. Lay the person down and elevate the legs about 30 cm.
- If the burn is causing pain, cool with poured water. It is imperative that you keep the casualty warm. Remember, cool the burn, not the casualty.
- Do not puncture any blisters (they offer an infection-free cover) or remove pieces of tissue from the burned skin.
- Dress all burns with non-adhesive, absorbent dressings. Cling film can be laid across the burn to provide a non-stick, transparent dressing. Wrapping lengthways allows the area to swell without constriction.
- Call 999 immediately.

Chemical Burns

- Quickly flush the skin with large quantities of water if burned with liquid acids, alkalis, and caustic chemicals.
- Remove contaminated clothing to take any absorbed chemicals away from the skin. Do this while washing the casualty.

- Brush off a dry or solid chemical substance before flushing the skin with water. When a chemical agent gets wet, it becomes activated and will cause more damage to the skin than when it is dry.
- Apply water under very low pressure because pressure can drive the chemical deeper into the tissue.
- Do *not* attempt to neutralise a chemical because heat may be produced, resulting in more damage. Some product label directions for neutralising may be wrong. Save the container or label to get the name of the chemical.
- Call 999 immediately.
- If the chemical is in the eye, flush with more water than seems necessary (Figure 19). Use very low pressure. Remove any contact lenses.

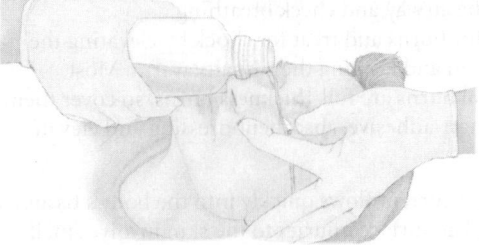

FIGURE 19 Immediately flush eye in case of chemical burns.

Electrical Injuries

Electrical Contact in Outdoor Situations

If electrical injury is caused by contact with a downed power line, the power must be turned off before a rescuer approaches anyone who may be in contact with the wire.

Leave cutting and disconnecting of wires to trained personnel with the proper equipment. Even material that does not usually conduct electricity, such as wood, may conduct high voltage. Prevent bystanders from entering the danger area.

Electrical Contact in Indoor Situations

When someone has incurred an electrical injury indoors, turn off the electricity at the circuit-breaker, fuse box, outside switch box, or unplug the appliance if the plug is undamaged. Do not touch the appliance or the casualty until the current is off.

Once the danger to rescuers has passed, first aid can begin.
- Open the airway and check breathing.
- Check for burns and treat for shock by elevating the legs 30 cm and keeping the casualty warm. Most electrical burns are full-thickness burns, so cover them with a non-adhesive, absorbent dressing and elevate the part.

Electrical current flows quickly into the body's tissues, then exits. The surface injuries to the skin involve small surface areas (entrance and exit points), and since clothing can be ignited by the electrical current, there may be heat burns as well. However, the major damage occurs deep under the skin.

All casualties of electrical shock should receive immediate medical care.

Frostbite

Frostbite results from exposure to sub-freezing temperatures. Damage occurs mainly to the feet, hands, ears, and nose.

Frostbitten parts are seldom re-warmed apart from at a medical facility because such facilities are usually nearby. If in a remote location, the *wet, rapid re-warming method* may be used and is preferred to slow re-warming, since the latter is associated with greater tissue damage.

Rapid Re-warming

- Do *not* re-warm if a medical facility is nearby or if there is any chance that the part may refreeze.
- Remove any clothing or constricting items that could impair blood circulation (eg, a ring).
- Put affected part(s) in warm (not hot) water. Water temperature should be around 40°C. If a thermometer is not available, test the water by sprinkling some over the inside of your arm. Maintain the water temperature by adding warm water as needed.
- Warming usually takes 20 to 40 minutes and should be continued until the tissues are soft and pliable.
- For ear or facial areas, apply warm, moist cloths and change them frequently.
- Do *not* break any blisters that may have formed.
- Do *not* rub the affected part.

Hypothermia

Hypothermia (cooling of the body core) can occur at temperatures above freezing as well as below it, particularly in cold, windy conditions or where the casualty is wet. In mild hypothermia, the casualty will be shivering.

Stop further heat loss by doing the following:
1. Get the casualty out of the cold environment.
2. Replace wet clothes with dry ones. Handle the casualty gently. Treat any injuries.
3. Add insulation beneath and around the casualty. Cover casualty's head, since 50% to 80% of the body's heat loss is through the head.
4. Seek medical care.

Heat-related Emergencies

Heatstroke
Signs and Symptoms
- Unresponsive
- Hot skin—may be dry or wet
- High body temperature
- Rapid pulse and breathing
- Weakness, dizziness, headache

First Aid

Heatstroke is a true emergency. If normal temperature is not quickly restored, the casualty could die or be permanently disabled.

- Move the casualty to a cool place. Remove heavy clothing; light clothing can be left in place.
- Immediately cool the casualty by any available means. Because ice is rarely available, an effective method is to wrap the casualty in wet towels or sheets, and fan him or her. Keep the cloths wet with cool water.

   Ice packs can also be placed on areas with abundant blood supply (eg, neck, armpits, and groin). Continue cooling the casualty until his or her condition improves. Stop at this point to prevent convulsions and hypothermia.

- Monitor breathing.
- If convulsions occur, care for them.
- *All heatstroke casualties need immediate medical care.*

Heat Exhaustion
Signs and Symptoms

- Heavy sweating
- Weakness
- Fast pulse
- Normal body temperature
- Headache and dizziness
- Nausea and vomiting

First Aid

- Move the casualty to a cool place.
- Keep casualty lying down with straight legs elevated 30 cm.
- Cool the casualty by applying cold packs or cold, wet towels or cloths. Fan the casualty.
- Give the casualty cool water or a sports drink if he or she is fully responsive.
- If no improvement is noted within 30 minutes, seek medical care.

Fractures

A fracture is a broken bone. In the more common closed fracture the skin is not cut (Figure 20A). In open fractures the overlying skin is lacerated (Figure 20B).

Signs and Symptoms

- **Deformity.** This is not always obvious, so always compare the injured part with the opposite, uninjured one.
- **Open wound.** Bone may be protruding.
- **Tenderness or pain.** The casualty usually can point to the site of pain. Pain is usually severe and constant and increases if the injured part is moved.
- **Swelling and discolouration.** Caused by bleeding from disrupted blood vessels. Initially, the area will be red, with bruises appearing several hours afterwards.
- **Loss of use.** The casualty cannot move or refuses to move the injured part. Sometimes movement is possible but produces severe pain.

FRACTURES

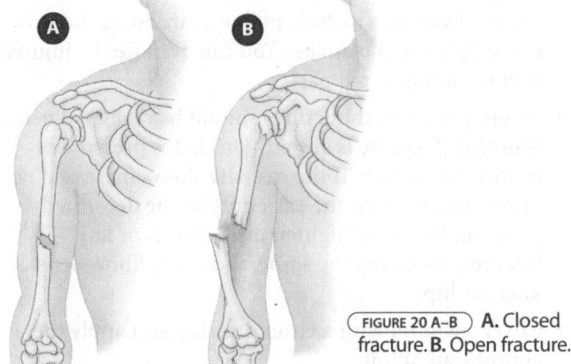

FIGURE 20 A–B   **A.** Closed fracture. **B.** Open fracture.

First Aid

- Treat for shock.
- Determine what happened and the location of the injury.
- Gently remove clothing covering the injury. Do *not* move the injured area unless necessary. Cut clothing at the seams if necessary.
- Control bleeding and cover all wounds before splinting. In dealing with open fractures, do *not* attempt to push bone ends back beneath the skin surface; cover them with a sterile dressing.
- If casualty's hand or foot on an injured extremity is cold, pale, and pulseless, seek immediate medical care.
- Splint all fractures before moving the casualty. Immobilise the joints above and below the injury site. Keep the fingers and toes exposed in order to check circulation.

- Many commonly available materials can be used as splints. Examples include pillows, cardboard, boards, newspapers, and blankets. You can even tie the injured part to an uninjured part.
- Severely deformed fractures should be realigned before splinting if a pulse is absent. This helps preserve or restore circulation. If the casualty shows increased pain or resistance, splint the extremity in the deformed position. Do *not* straighten dislocations or any fractures involving the spine, shoulder, elbow, wrist, knee, or hip.
- Cover a wound with a clean dressing and apply the appropriate splint.
- Stabilise the spine with rolled blankets or similar objects placed on either side of the neck and torso. In most cases it is best to wait until an ambulance arrives with trained personnel and proper equipment to handle spinal injuries. Tell the casualty not to move.
- To help control swelling and pain, use the RICE procedures found on pages 54–55.
- If in doubt, splint and treat as if there were a fracture.
- Seek medical care.

Dislocations

Dislocations occur when a joint comes apart and stays apart, with the bone ends no longer in contact.

Signs and Symptoms
- Similar to those of a fracture.

First Aid

- Check circulation, movement, and sensation of the injured extremity (compare with uninjured part).
- Splint as you would a broken bone. Use RICE procedures found on pages 54–55.
- Do *not* move the joint since nerve and blood vessel damage could occur.
- Seek medical care.

Splinting

Most bony injuries cause a lot of pain. One of the easiest ways of reducing the pain is to immobilise the affected area. Splinting stabilises broken bones and prevents any movement, resulting in a reduction of pain, bleeding, and tissue damage, and helps blood flow.

Whilst many commercially available splints are available, improvised devices often offer the same benefits. Whenever in doubt, splint.

Spinal Injuries

All *unresponsive casualties* should be treated initially as though they have spinal injuries. All *responsive casualties* sustaining severe injuries (eg, fall, diving incident, vehicle collision) should be carefully checked for spinal injuries before moving them. Head injuries serve as a clue, since the head may have been snapped suddenly in one or more directions, endangering the spine.

Other signs include numbness, tingling, or burning sensation in arms or legs, and inability to move arms and/or legs.

If there is doubt about a possible spinal injury, assume that the casualty has one until proven otherwise.

First Aid

- Check and monitor breathing. Do not use the head tilt–chin lift because it would move the neck.
- First aiders should normally wait for ambulance personnel to transport the casualty because their training and equipment may be necessary.
- Stabilise the casualty against any movement. Do *not* move the neck to reposition it. Only move the casualty when danger is present (eg, smoking or burning car or burning building). Bring help to the casualty, *not* the casualty to the help.
- Tell the casualty not to move. Place objects on either side of the head to prevent it from rolling from side to side.
- Casualties in water with potential neck or back injury must be floated gently to shore. Before removal from the water, the casualty must be secured to a longboard.

Muscle Injuries

Remember the initials R-I-C-E:

R = Rest. This means stop moving the injured part.
I = Ice. Methods of applying cold include using crushed ice as an ice pack or immersion in cold water. The application should continue for 10 minutes, three to four times during the first day, and if possible, the second day.

Place the ice or cold packs over the injured area. Constant use of an ice pack is not necessary because of the lasting effect of cold on body tissue.

C = Compression. Compression (elastic) bandage limits internal bleeding and should be worn continuously for 18 to 24 hours, but loosened at night.

Elastic bandages may be applied too tightly. Leave fingers and toes exposed so that changes in colour and temperature change may be seen. Other signs that an elastic bandage is too tight are pain, numbness, and tingling.

Placing a sock or other soft cloth around the injury beneath an elastic bandage applies compression to not only bone and tendon, but also soft tissues.

E = Elevation. Elevating the injured area above the heart or on the same level limits circulation to that area and helps control internal bleeding.

Heart Attack

The following signs and symptoms may indicate a possible heart attack:
- Uncomfortable pressure, fullness, squeezing, or pain in the centre of the chest lasting 2 minutes or longer. It may come and go.
- Pain may spread to either shoulder, the neck, the lower jaw, or either arm.
- Any or all of the following: weakness, dizziness, sweating, nausea, or shortness of breath.

Not all of these warning signs occur in every heart attack. Many casualties deny that they are having a heart attack. If you see some of these signs, however, don't wait to seek medical care. Loss of time can seriously increase the risk of major damage. Get help immediately!

First Aid

- If you are with someone experiencing the signs and symptoms of a heart attack, act immediately.
- Expect denial. It is normal for someone with chest discomfort to deny the possibility of something as serious as a heart attack. But don't take no for an answer. Insist on taking prompt action.
- Call 999; however if you are in a remote area, consider driving to the nearest A&E department offering 24-hour emergency cardiac care. If possible, bring a mobile phone to call for help if the situation worsens along the way.

Knowing these things, you should also:

- Remain calm and provide plenty of reassurance to the casualty.
- Help the casualty to get into the most comfortable position they can. Loosen tight clothing.
- If your local guidelines allow, help the casualty to take an aspirin. If they have their own GTN (either tablet or spray), help them to take it. GTN helps relieve the pain of angina pectoris by widening the coronary arteries, thus supplying more oxygenated blood to the heart muscle.
- If the casualty becomes unresponsive, open the airway and check breathing. Start CPR if necessary.

Stroke

Signs and symptoms of a stroke depend on the area of the brain involved:
- Sudden weakness or numbness of the face, arm, and leg on one side of the body.
- Loss of speech, or trouble talking or understanding speech.
- Dimness or loss of vision, particularly in only one eye.
- Unequal pupils.
- Unexplained dizziness, unsteadiness, or sudden falls.
- Sudden severe headache.
- Loss of bladder and/or bowel control.

About 10% of strokes are preceded by "mini strokes" (**transient ischaemic attacks** or **TIAs**). TIAs are extremely important warning signs for stroke. TIA symptoms are very similar to those of a fully fledged stroke, but may resolve. Do *not* ignore TIAs; get medical care immediately.

First Aid

- Check and monitor the casualty's breathing. Provide CPR if needed.
- If the casualty is unresponsive, place him or her on one side, preferably with the paralysed side down. This position frees the casualty's useful extremities. Cushion the paralysed side. Positioning on the side permits secretions and vomit to drain into the cheek or out of the mouth rather than down the throat.

- Keep the responsive casualty in a supine position, with the upper body and head slightly elevated to allow for less blood pressure on the brain.
- Remove dentures and any mucus and food from the mouth in a swabbing motion with a piece of cloth wrapped around a finger.
- Do *not* give any liquids—the throat may be paralysed, which restricts swallowing.
- Seek immediate medical care and provide calm reassurance to the casualty and their family members.

Diabetic Emergencies

The most common diabetic emergency encountered is where the casualty's blood sugar level is very low, known as hypoglycaemia.

The signs and symptoms of hypoglycaemia are similar to those for conditions such as intoxication, poisoning, or concussion. It is recommended that if you are unsure of the casualty's underlying condition, err on the side of caution and treat as if they are hypoglycaemic.

- If the casualty is conscious, get them into a comfortable position and help them to take a sugary drink or sweet snack. If they start to respond, allow them to increase their food or drink intake until they recover.
- If the casualty is unresponsive, do not place anything in their mouth. Open the airway, check breathing, and place them in the recovery position or start CPR if necessary. Dial 999 immediately.

Convulsion

A simple convulsion is not necessarily a medical emergency. However, it can be a very frightening event for those witnessing one for the first time. A lot of convulsions will stop after a few minutes, allowing the casualty to recover without any ill effects.

For those dealing with someone who is having a convulsion:
- Cushion their head with something soft (eg, coat, blanket). Do not hold their head tightly or try to hold the casualty down. If you are in a confined space, try padding the area around the casualty.
- The casualty's airway will often be clenched shut. Do not try to open or place anything in their mouth during the convulsion.
- Loosen any tight clothing and continue to reassure the casualty throughout their convulsion.

When dealing with a casualty who is recovering immediately after a convulsion:
- Turn the casualty onto their side to allow secretions to drain out of the mouth.
- Loosen any tight clothing. Look for a MedicAlert bracelet.
- Sometimes people having convulsions may lose control of their bladder or bowel. Make every attempt to cover the casualty over whilst they recover, and continue to provide reassurance.

For an adult who is having a convulsion, call 999 when:
- This is the first time it has happened.
- The convulsion lasts more than 5 minutes.
- You cannot locate a MedicAlert bracelet on an unresponsive casualty.
- They recover slowly, have a second convulsion, or have difficulty breathing.
- There are signs of injury or illness.
- The patient is pregnant.

For a child who is having a convulsion, call 999 immediately.

Positional Asphyxia

Positional asphyxia occurs when the position of a casualty interferes with the normal mechanics of respiration, in essence stopping them from breathing adequately.

It is caused by an abnormal position of the body that interferes with the normal movements of inspiration and expiration. If anything inhibits this "mechanical" movement, air cannot move in or out of the lungs. By positioning a person in the prone (face down) position for lengths of time, or by applying weight to a prone person's back or any pressure to the neck area, the chest will not be able to expand and the person will struggle to breathe, causing positional asphyxia.

People likely to suffer from positional asphyxia include those who are suffering from:
- Current cardiac or respiratory health problems.
- Obesity.
- Physical exhaustion (especially following pursuit or a struggle).
- Stimulant intoxication (eg, cocaine).

Signs that a person is suffering from positional asphyxia include:

- Person is struggling to breathe
- Person becomes panicked
- Discolouration of the face/neck
- Neck veins become engorged
- Person states "I cannot breathe"
- Person becomes limp/unresponsive
- Person appears to have stopped breathing.

If a person starts to display any of the above, you must either release or modify any restraint as far as reasonably practicable. Medical support should be summoned where possible.

Emergency Delivery of a Baby

In most cases, labour (the process of delivering a baby) begins slowly and women have plenty of time to get to a hospital, but occasionally delivery must occur without medical care. Most deliveries progress normally. Care should focus on helping the mother accomplish this natural process. Labour begins with contractions of the muscle of the uterus (the womb), causing a cramping sensation in the abdomen. The contractions become more frequent as labour progresses. Signs that delivery may occur too soon to allow transport to the hospital include:

- Contractions occurring less than 1 minute apart.
- Mother feels the need to push or move her bowels.
- Top of baby's head (or other body part) is visible.

If you do not believe there is enough time to safely transport the mother to hospital, make preparations for delivery:

- Call 999.
- Assist the mother to a comfortable position (usually lying down or squatting).
- Prepare a clean area for the mother to lie on. Expect a fair amount of blood and fluid, so place absorbent towels or pads under her, if possible.
- Wash your hands. Wear medical gloves if available.
- Avoid touching the vaginal area, and never put anything into the vagina.
- Always explain what you are doing.

Once the baby starts to come out:

- Have the mother stop pushing, so the baby does not come out too fast.
- Support the baby's head.
- Remove any membrane that may be covering the baby's face.
- If the umbilical cord is around the baby's neck, unloop it.
- If a part of the baby other than the head (like the arm or leg) comes out first, do not try to deliver the baby. Await the ambulance service and place the mother on her left side if possible.
- Mothers frequently pass some stool. Wipe it away from the vagina and baby using a clean cloth or gauze pad.

Once the baby is out:

- Hold the baby with the head down slightly, to allow fluids to drain from the mouth and nose.
- Dry the baby and wrap in something clean and dry to keep the baby warm.

EMERGENCY DELIVERY OF A BABY

- Tap or rub the baby to stimulate breathing.
- If the baby does not start breathing or crying within a few seconds, begin CPR.

If the ambulance service is not present yet, begin aftercare:
- If possible, keep the baby lower than the mother's abdomen to allow blood to drain into the baby.
- Give baby to mother to hold.
- If bleeding does not slow, treat for shock.
- Delivery of the placenta (afterbirth) usually occurs within 30 minutes. Save any tissue and send with the mother to hospital.

Quick Emergency Index

A
Abdominal injuries, 5, 34
Adult CPR, 8–10
AED model, 15
AIDS, 24
Allergic reactions
  to Elastoplast, 25
  insect, 38
Amputation, 22–23

B
Baby, emergency delivery of, 61–63
Bandages, 23, 25
Basic Life Support (BLS)
  adult CPR, 8–10
  AED, 15
  child CPR, 12–14
  choking, 9, 11–12
  defined, 7
  infant CPR, 14–15
  recovery position, 15–16
Bites
  animal, 23–25
  exotic animal, 38–39
  human, 23–25
  insect, 37–38
  to lips or tongue, 32
  tick, 39
Bleeding and wounds, 19–25
  amputation, 22–23
  bandaging, 23, 25
  bites, 23–25, 37–39
  head, 26
  overview of, 19–22
  physical examination of, 4
  sucking chest, 33–34
Blisters
  frostbite, 47
  overview of, 35–36
Burns
  chemical, 44–45
  electrical, 46
  flash, 30
  thermal, 42–44

C
Carbon monoxide, 40–42
Cardiopulmonary resuscitation (CPR)
  adult, 8–9
  AED, 15
  child, 12–14
  defined, 7
  infant, 14–15
  recovery position, 15–16
Casualty assessment
  chain of survival, 5–7
  initial check, 3–4
  physical examination, 4–5
  SAMPLE history, 5–6
Chemicals
  burns from, 29–30, 44–45
  incapacitant spray exposure, 41–42
Chest injuries, 33–34
  physical examination of, 4
Child CPR, 12–14
Choking
  in adult, 11–12
  signs and symptoms, 9–11
Cold injuries, 47–48
Compression injuries, 26
Concussion, 26
Convulsions, 59–61

D
Dental injuries, 31–33
Diabetic emergencies, 58
Dislocations, 52–53
Dressings, 23, 25

E
Electrical injuries, 45–46
Examination, victim, 3–7
Exposure
  frostbite, 47
  hypothermia, 48
  incapacitant spray, 41–42
Eye injuries
  blows, 29
  chemical burns, 29–30, 45
  cuts, 29